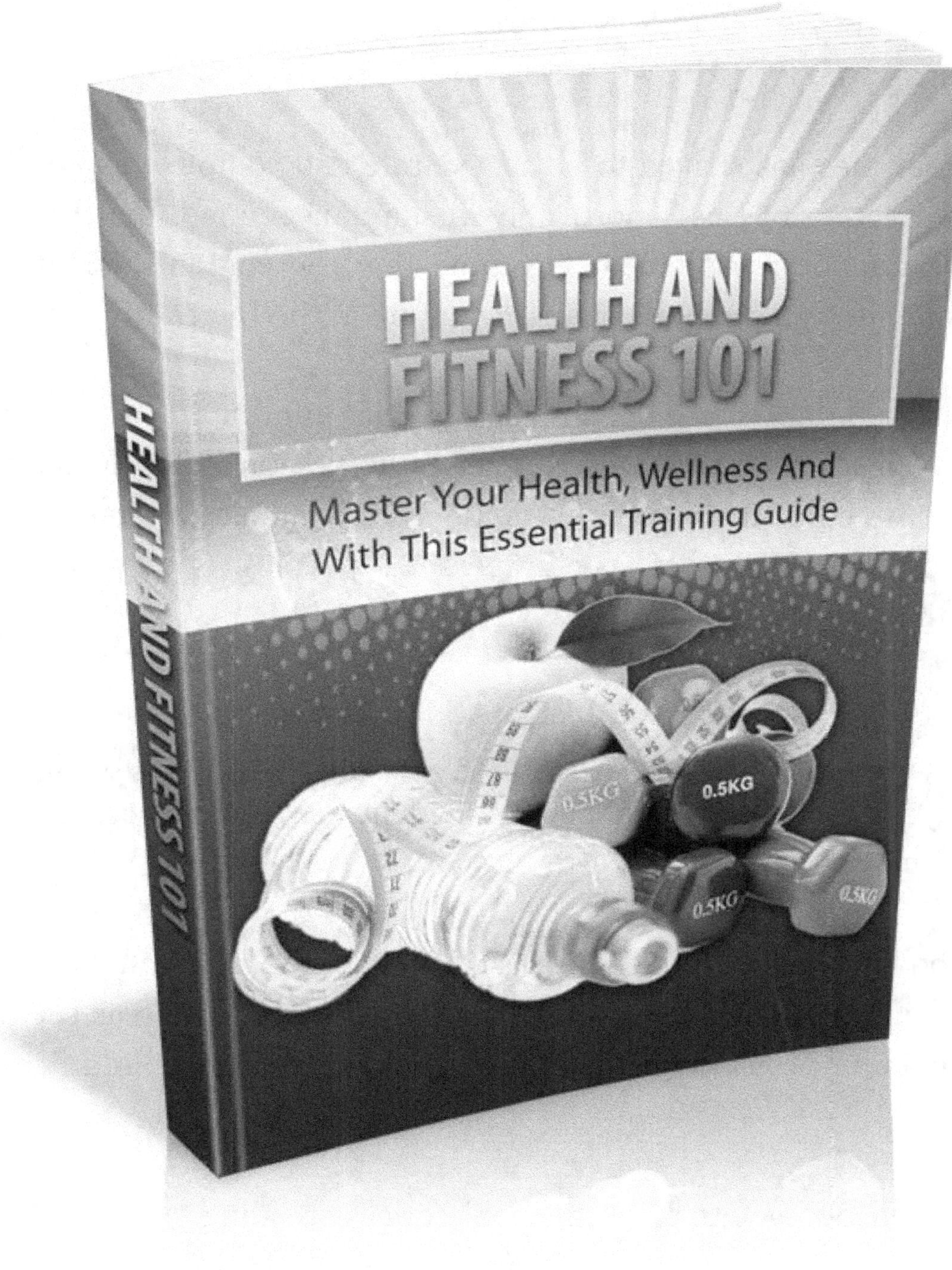

HEALTH AND FITNESS 101

Master Your Health, Wellness And With This Essential Training Guide

Terms and Conditions
LEGAL NOTICE

Table Of Contents

Foreword

Self-improvement is a thing which you must practice throughout your life because once you started to believe that you are perfect then, things will start to become complex. You need to know that no one is perfect and no one can be perfect.

There is always room for some improvements whether it is in your personality, in your health, in your fitness or in any other thing but you should keep trying for the better state. There are hundreds of therapies which help you to get rid of all kinds of mental stress and once you are relieved mentally then, you can always feel better in every part of your life.

In this EBook, I will guide you for some healthy living style and will tell you that how can you improve your physical fitness and get rid of different health problems which keep bothering you.

This will be a very smooth ride and you will enjoy reading every word of this EBook. I am going to tell you very basic stuff which you must have heard but you never gave attention to these things.

You need to pay close attention, in order to improve your fitness level. You may have read different books, in order to get rid of some health problem but with this EBook you are guaranteed to find solution of almost every health problem.

If you keep acting upon things mentioned in this EBook then, there is no reason that your health and fitness level will not improve.

There is no medication advertised or mentioned in this EBook because for any kinds of medicine, you always need to consult your doctor and I do not want to get people in trouble by telling them some random medicine.

Everything is based upon natural method and there are tips which can improve your whole daily life and will turn your unhealthy life style into a very healthy and productive life style. So keep reading the EBook till end and enjoy your improved health!

Health And Fitness 101

Master Your Health, Wellness And Fitness With This Essential Training Guide

Chapter 1:

Analyze and Change Your Lifestyle into A Healthier One

Synopsis

If you are living your life without any clue about your work routine and its effects on your health and fitness then, this chapter is definitely for you.

- ❖ Lack of physical activity
- ❖ Control your weight with little extra movement
- ❖ Check your eating habits

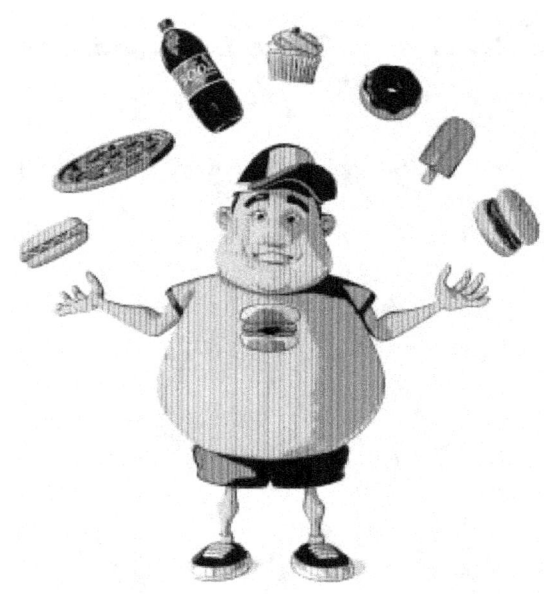

Have A Look

In modern times, life is very tough and competitive. You have to work hard, in order to stay in this society and in this hectic work routine, you often forget to take care of yourself. I have seen people who work for more than 12-15 hours a day and still they feel unsatisfied with their work. In this kind of life style, there are so many glitches which you can fix to optimize your routine.

These glitches are also not very hard to find and with very little attention, you can get them and repair them easily. You must have heard this too often that you should live a healthy life style but have you ever thought what actually a healthy life style is. Is it just about not smoking, doing exercise and keeping your weight under control? This formula sounds simple but believe it or not, it takes some time and hard work to be implemented in real life.

If you do not exercise, and your eating habits are also unstable then, it will take very small steps to bring you on track. You just need to make some very slight adjustments in your daily life style and these adjustments will make your life healthier and fit.

Lack of Physical Activity

Biggest drawback of modern office life is lack of physical activity. You have to sit in your chair throughout the day and after a tiring day in office, you go to your home and after taking your dinner you cannot even walk and go to sleep. This is very dull and unhealthy routine but you can make it little more energetic for you and that will also not get too much attention or time from you. You can just get up 20-30 minutes early than you do now and go out for a short walk.

Even if you think that is not possible for you then, you can just take bus to your office instead of your car. This will add some walk in your routine. This much movement and activity can be so much advantageous for you that it can save you from lots of heart diseases as well it will improve your respiration and will make you feel your weight. Your joint stability will get improve and you will be flexible enough according to your age. It will also help you in reducing anxiety and depression and will improve your mood and you will be able to work with more concentration. Smaller movement schemes like gardening on weekends, daily walk and similar other activities can also help you to control your weight.

Control Your Weight with Little Extra Movement

There are some very simple and basic things which you can do to make your life more active and to increase your physical activities. It is not necessary that you pay heavy gym fees to exercise and to do proper weight loss instead if your weight is not alarmingly high and you just want to control it then, you can do it by adding some simple thing like you can go out for a walk daily with your family instead of just sitting on the couch and watching TV. No matter that walk is to your local grocery store but it will be lot more active task than just sitting on the couch. Walk is a very important aspect which can help you to reduce and control your weight. There are so many ways which can add some walk in your life for example instead of going to the mall in your car, take a walk, take your dog for some extra outing in nearby park and similar other things can be very healthy for you.

Some people and especially men have this habit of not doing any home chores. This is also an unhealthy life style because house chores like gardening, some light cooking and other similar things which you can do in your weekends are very healthy activities and these activities will increase the physical work out.

These chores will also give you a chance to facilitate your partner and she will feel very happy as you are helping her in her work. Best way to add physical activities in your daily routine is to make a list of everything which you do in one day and analyze that list. If you find yourself sitting around too much then, try and look for some alternate time where you can add some physical activity.

Check Your Eating Habits

Eating is another thing which can impact a lot on your daily life and especially on your weight management. A healthy diet plan can always keep your weight in check and if you are eating without any certain plan then, it will create chaos for your body and will ultimately increase or decrease your weight alarmingly. You need to know that how many calories you are consuming every day. There are lots of different calories meters available which can tell you the exact amount of calories in your daily diet. Following are some of the general trends which you can follow to make your diet plan healthier.

First of all, you need to add more fruit in your diet. Fruit is the healthiest natural diet which you can get and almost every fruit is enriched with different vitamins and these vitamins are available in their purest form in these fruits.

These days, people are very afraid of vegetables and they do not like to add vegetables in their diet because vegetables are not very spicy but you should not be a victim of this trend as it is a very unhealthy trend and you need to add good amount of vegetables in your diet.

Even if you do not like to take vegetables in their traditional form then, add them in some snacks and eat them every now and them with lunch or dinner. You should also try and add a salad with your dinner and lunch.

This is a very healthy habit which can make you to cut your appetite and you will be eating healthier food. Cut the use of fat and try to use some fat free dairy. Try to avoid junk and fast food as much as you can because it is very unhealthy food with full of unhealthy fats.

Chapter 2:

Secrets of Health and Fitness

Synopsis

I will tell you some secret ways of boosting your health and being fit.

- ❖ Healthy eating
- ❖ Regular exercise
- ❖ Stress management
- ❖ Alternate health and medicine options
- ❖ Sleep well

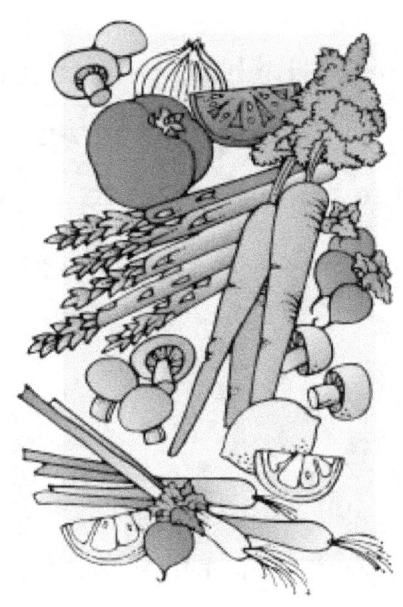

What's Behind It

First of all, you need to know that, in order to achieve a healthy and fit life, you must be living a very healthy life with proper and healthy life style. There are some very important ingredients in making your life fit and healthy and without those ingredients; you will not be able to get that precise health and fitness.

Most of the people think that without adapting to a certain tasteless diet plan and working hard in gym, they cannot get a healthy and fit life but this is not entirely true. Although doing exercise and keeping your diet healthy is important but this is not everything which you have to do for maintaining your health.

There are some other secrets which you must know and these secrets are also very easy to implement and execute. No matter how busy your life is but you can always find some time to execute these things which I am going to tell you now.

Healthy Eating

This is well-heard word which almost every person tells you that to get a health and fit body, you need to control your eating habits and make it healthier but no one tells you some easy way to do that. When it comes to healthy eating then, it does not just include eating healthier food but it also includes avoid eating all the unhealthy stuff.

You need to add natural elements like vegetables, fruit, unsaturated fat and unrefined carbohydrates. In start you will find it difficult to integrate these things in your diet plan but with time, you will learn about nutrition values of different diets and it will become lot easier for you to pick up the best diet plan. You should avoid eating junk and fast food because these food items contain unhealthy fat, refined carbohydrates and other similar things which can be very unhealthy and can increase your weight a lot.

Regular Exercise

Another very important thing which is exercise and you must include some sort of exercise in your daily routine. Some people have this misconception that only after joining a gym and paying heavy fee for that gym will give them proper work out routine but this is not necessary and secondly, people do not have that much time these days to go to gym daily. Office routines are very tough and to survive and make it work, you need to work more than 12 hours a day.

You need to find some alternate to that gym. You can add some light walk and jogging either in the evening or you can get up 25-30 minutes earlier than routine and go out for a walk. You can also add some walk in your routine by minimizing the use of car. You often use car for going to grocery store as well as to other routine places but you can avoid that car and go on your foot.

Stress Management

Being stress free is another thing which can give very positive effects in your life. Hectic work routine and no relaxing time can increase the stress level a lot and in lots of cases I have seen people going through sleeping disorder due to this constant stress. To avoid this stress and to minimize its effects, you can adopt some relaxation exercise like yoga or you can option for a massage after every 2-3 weeks.

These methods will help you a lot in decreasing the effects of stress and will make your life peaceful and stress free. When you are less tense then, you will be able to concentrate even more on your work and will increase your overall productivity.

Alternate Health and Medicine Options

Traditional doctors and medicines also have some side effects on your health and you should avoid them as much as possible. If you happen to be suffering from some minor health problems like temperature, flue and other similar problems then, you should not look for more traditional anti biotic instead look for some unorthodox medicines and look for side effect free medicines like homeopathic, massage therapy and other similar methods.

These methods will not also get you rid of that health problem but these are also made from totally natural elements which make them even healthier for your body. In other alternate medicine options you can look for herbal medicine, massage therapy, meditation, Ayurveda, reflexology, aromatherapy.

Sleep Well

Sleeping is another very important aspect of your life and it is the basic thing which helps your body and brain to relax and get ready for work. If you experience problem in getting a good and proper sleep then, you must do something to make this state better because I have seen people going half mad just because they cannot get proper sleep. In order to make your sleep more proper and better, you need to make sure that you are not taking your work to your bed. Make sure that before going to bed, you have solved all of your office and work problems and even if there is something left then, forget about it for the night and concentrate on getting a god sleep.

To implement all of the above things in your life, you need to make your life disciplined in first place. You need to make a commitment with yourself that you are going to make your life better and then follow that commitment to your fullest effort.

Some people try to adopt such schemes as proper diet plan, proper exercise plan but they tend to execute it just for very small period of time. This is also not very effective because you need to be very consistent for proper results. This is the reason that I have described some very easy to adopt things which you can continue doing no matter what your daily life is.

Chapter 3:
Healthy Nutrition and Its Benefits

Synopsis

You will come to know the importance of healthy nutrition and its benefits in this chapter.

- ❖ Understanding nutrition
- ❖ Relationship between food, health and nutrition
- ❖ Guidelines for proper and healthy nutritional food

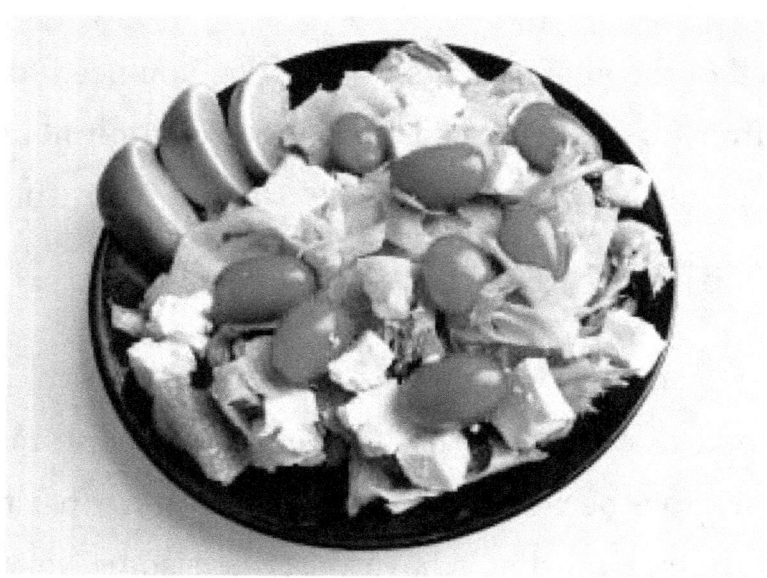

Nutrients

You would have heard lots of people saying that healthy nutrition is important for a healthy body but you need to know that is the actual meaning of healthy nutrition and why it is so important. Let's define nutrition.

"Nutrition is the process of giving your body all the important and necessary elements which can help it to grow in proper and balanced way." This is the simplest definition which tells you that you need to get proper food and proper diet which can help your body to grow in a better way. Healthy nutrition can make your body strong and can help it to grow and repair itself while an unhealthy nutrition plan can make your body weaker and can make you ill and you will not be able to fight against certain minor diseases.

Understanding Nutrition

The purpose of nutrition is quiet simple to understand and there are three things which can tell you its importance and purpose. First of all, you have a body and secondly that body needs some very precise things to nourish and to grow. Thirdly nutrition includes all those things which can help your body to grow. Now after this understanding, you need to know that what actual relationship of food and nutrition is. First of all, make this fact concrete that food and nutrition are not same things and there is some difference present between both of these.

Every food has not got nutrition and degree of nutrition in every food can vary. It may happen that some food items may contain high percentage of nutrition while some food items may not contain any nutrition at all. For example an apple can provide your body lot more nutrition than a doughnut. You can make it more interesting by understanding that when an apple goes in your system then it breaks down in substance which your body uses for growth and blood production but when you eat a doughnut then, your digestion system will say "hmm, I do not need much of this stuff, so, either throw it away or store it somewhere like in butt cheeks."

Relationship between Food, Health And Nutrition

Food, health and nutrition all are very closely related. The food which you eat can be either full of nutrition or it can not contain any nutrition. The nutrition which you provide to your body affects your health directly. The basic goal of everyone is to improve health and to improve health, you must provide enough and adequate amount of nutrition to your body and especially for your physical health and fitness, you must make sure that you are providing enough nutrition to your body. There are four categories in nutrition which your body always need in enough amounts. These four categories are protein, fat, carbohydrate and vitamins. You need to make sure that the food which you are eating contains necessary amount of these elements and if you observe all the processed food then, you will know that all of these are labeled with their nutrition values and these labels are there for you to make an informed choice about your nutritional needs.

Guidelines for Proper And Healthy Nutritional Food

In order to provide your body with proper nutritional elements, you need to follow these very simple food guidelines and these will help you to make better choice of food. You should have a general idea of healthy and unhealthy food in first place and this idea will allow you to choose healthier food without going through lists of food items.

Every food which can be metabolized means that can be converted into substance which is needed to grow is healthy food. You can make a measuring foot which can tell you the health value of a particular food item. Make it in three parts and first of all think about those foods which are totally processed and baked as these foods have almost zero natural elements in them like doughnuts, fast food and other similar items. These foods have absolute nutritional value and in most of the cases they are found to be harmful for your body. Second are those food which are cooked with natural ingredients like meat, chicken, vegetables and similar other items. These foods are nutritional to some extent because they contain natural elements and you can add these food items in your regular diet. Third are the food items which are totally natural and have no preservatives and other similar things added like fruits, fresh juice, milk and other similar items. These are the items which carry most nutritional value.

Chapter 4:

Stress Management and Your Health

Synopsis

In this chapter, I will tell you that how important it is to be stress free for a healthier life.

- ❖ Stress relief
- ❖ Relaxation techniques
- ❖ Progressive relaxation
- ❖ Breathing relaxation
- ❖ Yoga and other relaxing exercises

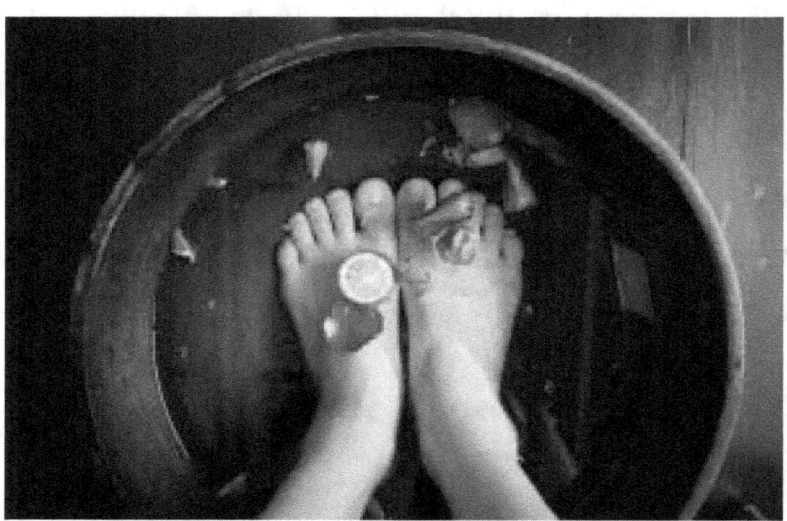

Tension

Stress is a normal psychological response of your body to ever increasing and ever demanding life. These days, our life is so tough that we have to suffer from stress and anxiety almost every day. According to a survey most of the Americans go through stress and anxiety at some point during the year.

There are endless reasons for this stress but your need to know that our brain is a very delicate part of our body and whenever it faces a situation which he cannot consume or solve then, it releases a response for the whole body to release hormones which control that situation but unfortunately these days, this call for hormones is coming throughout the year and ultimately you cannot feel the relaxed state which comes after the release of hormones. To ensure that you do go in that relaxed state, you need to make sure that you are going through proper stress management. If you do not do anything about your stress then, most likely your body will never find that relaxing state and that can lead to some fatal diseases.

Stress Relief

These days, almost everyone is stressed out and there are endless reasons behind this stress but you need to do proper stress management to make your life better and peaceful. There is very fixed procedure for stress relief in which at first you have to identify your stress trigger. This trigger can be of any type. Usual triggers are relationship pressure, financial losses, family pressure and other similar things.

Positive events can also trigger stress for example if you are married and you started a new job ad bought a new house in single year then, you can be stressed out due to too much attention and financial pressure. Negative events are always bigger causes of stress but once you have identified your right stress trigger then, you need to rectify that triggering point.

Sometimes removing these triggers can be as easy as turning off your TV when evening news are too stressful but sometimes it can be difficult enough to make you go through some proper health care. There are different stress relief strategies being implemented by people and you can try more than one strategy and see the results on yourself. Most of these strategies are natural and do not involve much of medication but some can ask you to take some mild medication.

Relaxation Techniques

Relaxation techniques are a very effective method to rectify stress from your life. There are lots of relaxation techniques available and following are some of the most popular ones.

Progressive Relaxation

This is very common and very effective types of relaxation techniques. You do not need to go to some professional therapist for this technique and can implement this technique perfectly at your house. You just need to relax in your bed, sofa or couch where ever you feel most relaxed. Lie down, close your eyes and experience all the stressful events and try to make them go from your mind. Concentrate hard on your present state and try to relax as much as you can. Inhale and exhale longer breaths and make sure that you have no distraction around like kids, TV or any other thing. Do this for more than 10 minutes and after doing this, you will feel pretty relaxed and calm.

Breathing Relaxation

There are lots of breathing techniques which are also known as relaxation techniques but these techniques are little difficult to learn you need to consult some professional therapist to learn them. You just need 2-3 sessions with your therapist to learn these breathing and relaxing exercises. Once you learn them, then, you will feel a very positive change in your stress level and you will be able to control your stress and anxiety.

Yoga and Other Relaxing Exercises

There are different exercises which can also help you to relax and especially if you start practicing yoga then, you will know that these exercises give you control over your emotions and feeling too. To learn these exercises, it is important that you find some professional trainer who can guide you for the right procedure because doing them improperly will not give you much benefit and will be just a waste of your time and money.

Some Unorthodox Techniques

If you find all of the above techniques and exercise plans boring and hard then, you need to turn towards some more unorthodox exercise or you should say relaxing plans. Massaging is very important and very effective relaxing therapy which can get rid of whole your tension and stress. There are different massaging techniques which you can apply but you should avoid doing it too often and keep this for just once or twice in a month. Other than massaging, if you have too much stress and you do not know any way out of that stress and anxiety then, you should go for some more particular and professional therapies like psychotherapy. There are some negative concepts about this therapy but you should know that it is totally harmless and is just for mental and stress control.

All of the above mentioned methods are effective and they are proved to be effective because hundreds and thousands of people have tried them and found positive results out of them. If you have executed one of these methods and have not found the required result then, this means that that particular method was not suited to your needs and you need to adopt another more suitable. Every method has certain limitations and certain methods are suited in certain situations. You should give the choice of method to your doctor or therapist because they will analyze your problem more deeply and will prescribe the most suited method.

Chapter 5:
Exercise and Its Type

Synopsis

In this chapter, I will tell you about different types of exercises and their effects on different aspects of your life and health.

- ❖ Exercise to improve bone and muscle strength
- ❖ Flexibility increasing exercises
- ❖ Cardiovascular exercise
- ❖ Aerobics

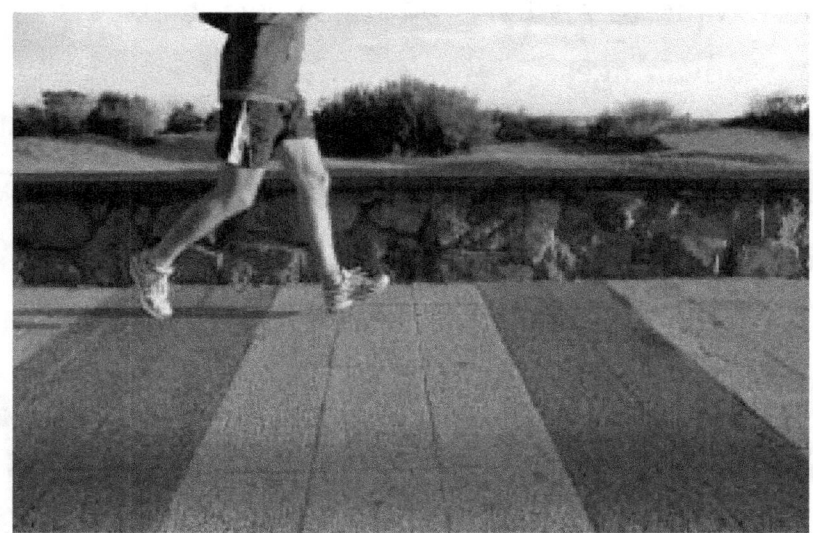

Get Moving

If someone has told you that only a hard and tough exercise routine can make you healthy then, he has misguided you completely because although exercise is necessary for your health and fitness but it is not necessary that you have to work out for more than an hour every day to stay fit. After hearing this kind of hard working plan, most of the people lose their heart and they think that they do not have time for this crap and they are better without it. This is also a wrong attitude and you should look for more proper and realistic guide. Obviously, you have a busy life routine and you cannot get time for exercise daily but you can obviously find 15-20 minutes daily for very relaxing kinds of exercises which can help you to get rid of whole day's stress and can make your fresh for a new start. In this discussion, I am going to give you all those secret exercise types and will also tell you their advantages.

First of all, you need to know that there are four kinds of exercise plans which are available and all four of them have different advantages for your physical health.

Exercise To Improve Bone and Muscle Strength

These exercises are also called strength and resistance increasing exercises. Most of the people take body building as strength and resistance increasing exercise but you need to know that body building is another category of exercise in which the primary goal of the person is to enhance muscle growth.

You can add some weight lifting and body building in your fat burning and weight control plan but you should do it to an extent where your body can bear it without any problem. If you over tried this exercise then, your whole body can be a mess. I have seen people joining gyms and doing hard exercise just by watching other people doing it. This is not the way to go instead consult your trainer personally and ask him about appropriate exercises which can fit in your needs. If your weight is under control and you need just light exercise to keep your healthy system going then, you do not need to lift heavy weights.

Flexibility Increasing Exercises

Second type of exercise plan can be to increase your flexibility and in more common terms you can say that if you used to have pain in your arms, legs, lower back, neck and other similar areas of your body then, you need to make your body more flexible. Flexibility will increase resistance and you will be able to cope with more difficult positions and postures easily. You have to go through different postures in daily life for example if you work in an office then, you can be given an uncomfortable chair at times or you may be given some work in which you have to concentrate hard on computer screen and you cannot rest your back with chair. In these situations, if you do not have any flexibility in your body then, it will create problems but regular flexibility exercises which will not take more than 10-15 minutes of your time, will increase this flexibility and will make you feel better and active.

Cardiovascular Exercise

Cardio means heart and vascular means the vessels of blood and this whole phrase means that these exercises improve the functionality of your lungs and make the use of oxygen more effective and rectify any heart problems which you can have. These exercises are little time consuming and should be properly learned from your doctor or trainer. Most of the times, people who already have got some heart problem perform these kinds of exercises to avoid any future problems.

Aerobics

Aerobics are the last type of exercises which are most helpful for maintaining a healthy body. These exercises are very simple and they do not need any special preparation and time frame for execution. If you just get up early in the morning and do some dancing then, this is also a type of aerobics but most of the aerobics are for young and energetic people as some difficult angels and twists are included in this exercise routine. You need to first learn this exercise from some professional trainer of aerobics and once you have learnt them then, these exercises will not require more than 10 minutes of your daily time.

Chapter 6:
Tips for Weaker and Old Age People

Synopsis

If you are a senior citizen and striving for good health then, this chapter will give you perfect ways to maintain a very fit and healthy body.

- ❖ Keep your mind young
- ❖ Some secret health tips for older people
- ❖ Regular health check ups
- ❖ Overcome your bad habits
- ❖ Senior safety at home

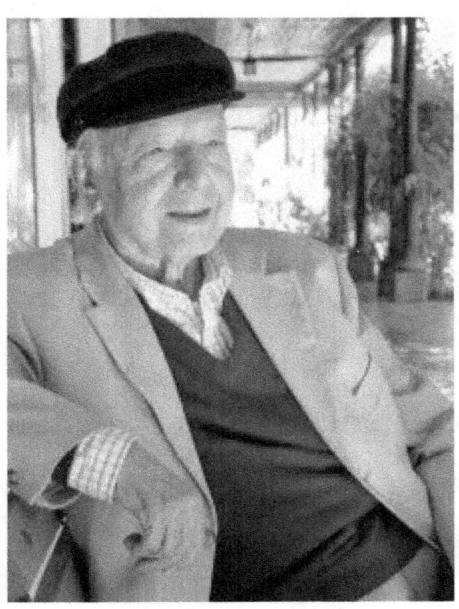

Seniors

Our body is just like a very delicate machine and more we use this machine, more sensitive it becomes to faults. Similar is the case with old age because in our old age, we had consumed almost everything of our body and it needs special care and extreme attention to stay fit and working 100 percent. If you are in your early 40's then, you should know that you are entering an age where very small diseases can over run you and you will be left helpless but there are lots of things which you can always do to improve your daily life and stay fit even in your old age.

Keep Your Mind Young

Most of the people get old because they think they are old. Your mind frame has a very deep effect on your overall health. You should never say to yourself that you have become old and weak because if you trusted this opinion then, it will make you even weaker and older.

You should keep your spirits up and say to yourself that it is not the time to lie down on your bed instead you should participate actively in daily activities. I have seen people who lie down on their bed when they enter in their 50's and have their grandkids. This is not the way instead you should remain active and try to participate in your family matters as it tells you your importance and you do not stick to that plan of being weaker.

Some Secret Health Tips for Older People

Regular exercise is the key to stay fit for any age group but the types of exercise keep changing. When you are young and youthful then, you can afford to do aerobics, weight lifting and other similar exercises but once you cross your 50 then, your bones and muscles become weaker and you cannot execute all of the those exercise plans.

You need to know this fact and choose some light and mild exercises for you like stretching, walking, light jogging and other similar exercises. Walk and jogging are two of the most essential and most effective exercises which you can do and these will help you to not only maintain your health but these will also help you to get rid of certain heart and lungs diseases.

You can also try light kinds of aerobics and other hard stretching exercise but try them for a particular period and see their effect. If you feel strain or pain in your muscles and weakness in your whole body then, you should know that these are not the appropriate exercises for you.

Regular Health Check Ups

As I mentioned above that in older age, your muscles, bones and other vital organs become weaker and they tend to get diseased and faulty very easily. So to avoid any unpleasant situation, you should have regular checkups from your doctor. These checkups will ensure that everything is working properly inside your body and even if something is going wrong, it will be diagnosed in early stages and doctors will be able to give you proper medication to cure it as soon as possible. There is no better person than your family doctor to do this checkup because he knows your history and he will know your problems much better than a new doctor.

Overcome Your Bad Habits

As we grow up, we develop certain bad habits like smoking, drinking and other similar things. These habits may not harm you mush in young age and you will be able to resist their side effects and bad effects on your health in that age but when you get into older age then, these habits can be life threatening for you.

Drinking disturbs your immune system is disturbed at that age and you are no longer resisting its side effects. It can destroy your digestion system and can initiate some very harmful liver diseases too. Similarly if you smoke too much then, it can damage your lungs. In order to make your last few years easy on yourself, you need to quit these habits and if you cannot quit them completely then, at least try to limit them.

Senior Safety At Home

In old age, people tend to fell sick a lot more often and it is necessary that they should be provided with proper support at home. Muscles become weak and sometime weakness becomes terrible and they cannot even walk properly.

In this state, they need to have proper support while climbing stairs and they should also have proper support in their bath rooms so that they do not slip from slippery tiles of bathroom. Going in an old age home is not a very good option because that place sucks from many points of view.

There is a very lonely feeling in these places which makes you very disturbed mentally. In last years of your life, you always need someone from your family and especially from your kids to help you out and to look after you. This gives you a very soothing and helping atmosphere if someone your love is always around to help you in your bad times.

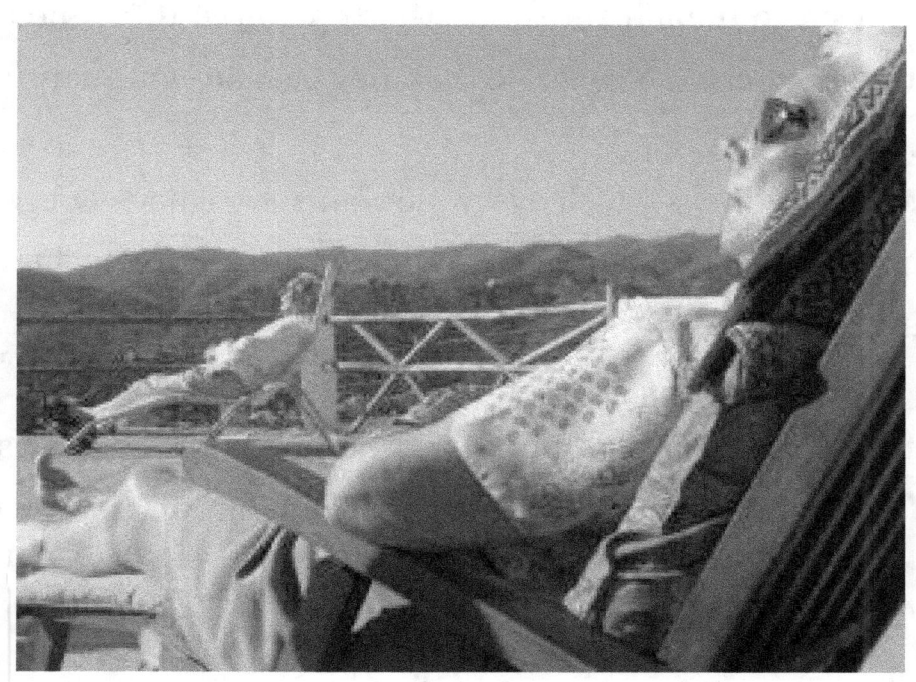

Wrapping up

After reading this whole EBook, I am hundred percent sure that you will be able to change your life style to a very healthy one. You need to understand the fact that people whom you see more active in their lives, successful and chasing their dreams, are also people just like you and me but they have altered their life course to be a more effective, health friendly and fit.

They have struggled hard to achieve that perfect life but once they get there then, it seems that everything was very easy for them. Consistency is the key to success in any field and similar is the case with your health and fitness. You need to implement some health patterns throughout your life and make those patterns so concrete that they become your nature.

There are so many things which everyone wants to achieve but people back down from their dreams just because they do not want to hard work to achieve that dream.

There is universal law of attraction that when you try to access something from pure heart and deep desire then, everything around you helps you to get to that thing.

This is true in everything and whether that is a very high post in your office or you have to lose weight and gain a beach body in less than 2 months, everything is possible. You just need to be sincere with yourself and do not cheat yourself about anything.

Once you start to be sincere with yourself and subtract all the lies from your personal life then, everything will become easy and you will be able to achieve everything.

After reading this whole EBook, if you find out that above mentioned tasks are too heavy and hard for you and you cannot change your life style then, this is not your acts but just thought of a lazy person who is not ready to give away some of his comforts for a progressive future. Overcome your fears and achieve a healthy and fit lifestyle.

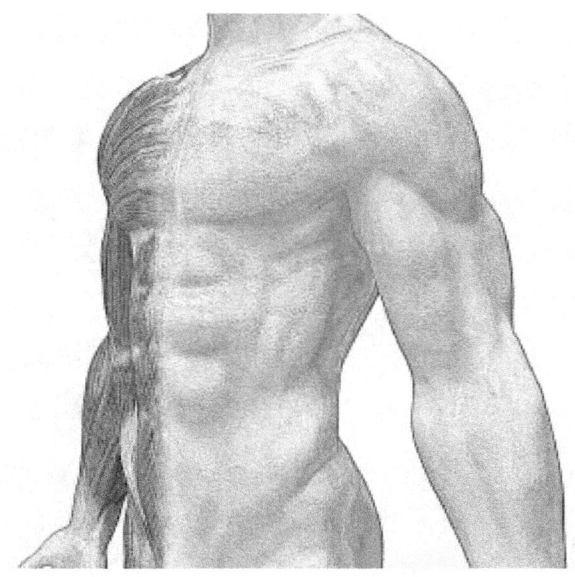